The Diabetic Cookbook for Beginners

*Simple, Quick and Easy Recipes
for a Healthy Lifestyle and Balanced Diet*

Sophie Kruis

© **Copyright 2021 By Sophie Kruis - All rights reserved.**

The content contained within this book may not be reproduced, duplicated or transmitted without direct written permission from the author or the publisher.

Under no circumstances will any blame or legal responsibility be held against the publisher, or author, for any damages, reparation, or monetary loss due to the information contained within this book. Either directly or indirectly.

Legal Notice:

This book is copyright protected. This book is only for personal use. You cannot amend, distribute, sell, use, quote or paraphrase any part, or the content within this book, without the consent of the author or publisher.

Disclaimer Notice:

Please note the information contained within this document is for educational and entertainment purposes only. All effort has been executed to present accurate, up to date, and reliable, complete information. No warranties of any kind are declared or implied. Readers acknowledge that the author is not engaging in the rendering of legal, financial, medical or professional advice. The content within this book has been derived from various sources. Please consult a licensed professional before attempting any techniques outlined in this book.

By reading this document, the reader agrees that under no circumstances is the author responsible for any losses, direct or indirect, which are incurred as a result of the use of information contained within this document, including, but not limited to, errors, omissions, or inaccuracies.

Table Of Contents

INTRODUCTION 7

BREAKFAST RECIPES 9
   1. Blueberry Breakfast Cake 9
   2. Whole-Grain Pancakes 12
   3. Buckwheat Grouts Breakfast Bowl 14
   4. Peach Muesli Bake 16
   5. Steel-Cut Oatmeal Bowl With Fruit And Nuts 18

APPETIZER RECIPES 21
   6. Cheesy Broccoli Bites 21
   7. Easy Caprese Skewers 23
   8. Grilled Tofu with Sesame Seeds 25
   9. Kale Chips 27
  10. Simple Deviled Eggs 29
  11. Sautéed Collard Greens and Cabbage 31
  12. Roasted Delicata Squash with Thyme 33

FIRST COURSE RECIPES 35
  13. Blueberry and Chicken Salad 35
  14. Beef and Red Bean Chili 37
  15. Berry Apple Cider 39
  16. Brunswick Stew 41

SECOND COURSE RECIPES 44
  17. Cauliflower Rice with Chicken 44
  18. Turkey with Fried Eggs 46
  19. Sweet Potato, Kale, and White Bean Stew 48
  20. Slow Cooker Two-Bean Sloppy Joes 50
  21. Lighter Eggplant Parmesan 52
  22. Coconut-Lentil Curry 55

SIDE DISH RECIPES 58
  23. Brussels Sprouts 58
  24. Garlic and Herb Carrots 60
  25. Cilantro Lime Drumsticks 62
  26. Eggplant Spread 64
  27. Carrot Hummus 66

- 28. Vegetable Rice Pilaf 68
- 29. Curry Roasted Cauliflower Florets 70

SOUPS & STEWS 73

- 30. Dill Celery Soup 73
- 31. Creamy Avocado-Broccoli Soup 75
- 32. Fresh Garden Vegetable Soup 77
- 33. Raw Some Gazpacho Soup 79
- 34. Alkaline Carrot Soup with Fresh Mushrooms 81

DESSERTS 84

- 35. Peanut Butter Cups 84
- 36. Fruit Pizza 85
- 37. Choco Peppermint Cake 87
- 38. Roasted Mango 89
- 39. Roasted Plums 90
- 40. Figs with Honey & Yogurt 91
- 41. Flourless Chocolate Cake 92
- 42. Lava Cake 94

JUICE AND SMOOTHIE RECIPES 97

- 43. Dandelion Avocado Smoothie 97
- 44. Amaranth Greens and Avocado Smoothie 98
- 45. Lettuce, Orange and Banana Smoothie 100
- 46. Delicious Elderberry Smoothie 102
- 47. Peaches Zucchini Smoothie 103
- 48. Ginger Orange and Strawberry Smoothie 104
- 49. Kale Parsley and Chia Seeds Detox Smoothie 106
- 50. Watermelon Limenade 108

CONCLUSION 110

Introduction

Diabetes is a condition where the body is no longer able to self-regulate blood glucose. When you eat a food that contains carbohydrates, the body breaks it down into sugar (also called glucose) during digestion. This glucose passes through the walls of the intestines into the blood, which causes blood sugar to rise.

In response, the pancreas secretes a hormone called insulin. The role of insulin is to lower the blood sugar back to normal levels. It does this by moving the sugar out of the blood and into the cells, where it is used for energy. Think of insulin as a key that unlocks the doors to the cells. But if you have diabetes, either the body doesn't make enough insulin, or the cells don't respond to the insulin. This causes the blood sugar to build up in the bloodstream, resulting in high blood sugar. Long-term elevated blood sugar levels can affect almost every system in the body. Health complications can include heart disease, stroke, kidney failure, nerve damage, eye damage, and blindness. This is why it is so important to work with your healthcare team to come up with the best treatment plan for you and for you to take the leading part in your plan by eating healthy, staying physically active, and losing weight if necessary.

People with diabetes often think they need to become strictly focused on avoiding sugar or carbohydrates and neglect to consider the nutritional quality of their diet. While it's true that carbohydrates have the greatest impact on blood sugar, it is the diet as a whole that contributes to health, weight management, and blood sugar control. Strictly limiting carbohydrates found in fruit and whole grains while eating a diet high in saturated fat and sodium will not promote optimal health.

It is especially important to follow a heart-healthy diet because your risk for heart disease can be four times greater when you have type 2 diabetes.

Focusing on healthy foods, portion control of carbohydrates, and losing weight if you are overweight are the three most important things you can do to manage type 2 diabetes from a nutritional standpoint.

Breakfast Recipes

1. Blueberry Breakfast Cake

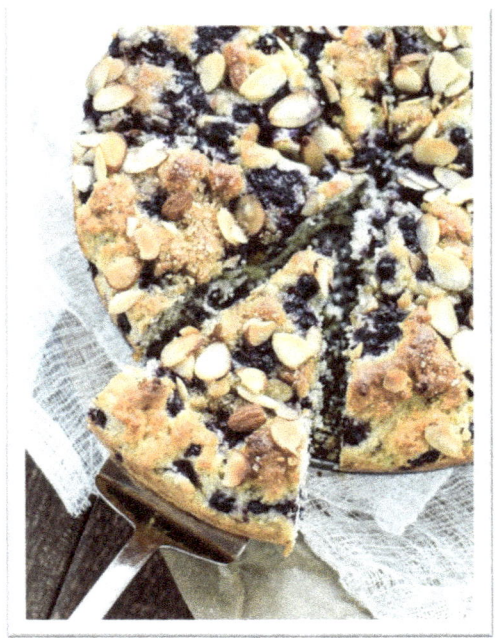

Preparation Time: 15 minutes

Cooking Time: 45 minutes

Servings: 12

Ingredients:

For the topping

- ¼ cup finely chopped walnuts
- 1/2 teaspoon ground cinnamon
- 2 tablespoons butter, chopped into small pieces

- 2 tablespoons sugar

For the cake
- Nonstick cooking spray
- 1 cup whole-wheat pastry flour
- 1 cup oat flour
- ¼ cup sugar
- 2 teaspoons baking powder
- 1 large egg, beaten
- 1/2 cup skim milk
- 2 tablespoons butter, melted
- 1 teaspoon grated lemon peel
- 2 cups fresh or frozen blueberries

Directions:

To make the topping
1. In a small bowl, stir together the walnuts, cinnamon, butter, and sugar. Set aside.

To make the cake
1. Preheat the oven to 350f. Spray a 9-inch square pan with cooking spray. Set aside.
2. In a large bowl, stir together the pastry flour, oat flour, sugar, and baking powder.

3. Add the egg, milk, butter, and lemon peel, and stir until there are no dry spots.
4. Stir in the blueberries, and gently mix until incorporated. Press the batter into the prepared pan, using a spoon to flatten it into the dish.
5. Sprinkle the topping over the cake.
6. Bake for 40 to 45 minutes, until a toothpick inserted into the cake comes out clean, and serve.

Nutrition: Calories: 177; Total Fat: 7g; Saturated Fat: 3g; Protein: 4g; Carbs: 26g; Sugar: 9g; Fiber: 3g; Cholesterol: 26mg; Sodium: 39mg

2. Whole-Grain Pancakes

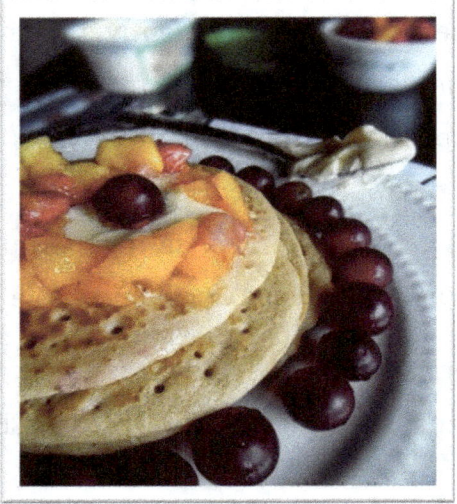

Preparation Time: 10 minutes

Cooking Time: 15 minutes

Servings: 4 to 6

Ingredients:

- 2 cups whole-wheat pastry flour
- 4 teaspoons baking powder
- 2 teaspoons ground cinnamon
- 1/2 teaspoon salt
- 2 cups skim milk, plus more as needed
- 2 large eggs
- 1 tablespoon honey

- Nonstick cooking spray
- Maple syrup, for serving
- Fresh fruit, for serving

Directions:
1. In a large bowl, stir together the flour, baking powder, cinnamon, and salt.
2. Add the milk, eggs, and honey, and stir well to combine. If needed, add more milk, 1 tablespoon at a time, until there are no dry spots and you have a pourable batter.
3. Heat a large skillet over medium-high heat, and spray it with cooking spray.
4. Using a ¼-cup measuring cup, scoop 2 or 3 pancakes into the skillet at a time. Cook for a couple of minutes, until bubbles form on the surface of the pancakes, flip, and cook for 1 to 2 minutes more, until golden brown and cooked through. Repeat with the remaining batter.
5. Serve topped with maple syrup or fresh fruit.

Nutrition: Calories: 392; Total Fat: 4g; Saturated Fat: 1g; Protein: 15g; Carbs: 71g; Sugar: 11g; Fiber: 9g; Cholesterol: 95mg; Sodium: 396mg

3. Buckwheat Grouts Breakfast Bowl

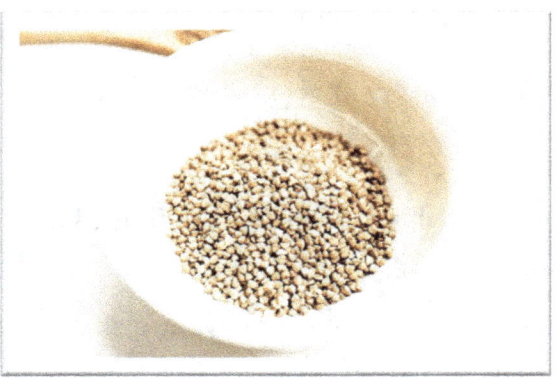

Preparation Time: 5 minutes, plus overnight to soak
Cooking Time: 10 to 12 minutes
Servings: 4
Ingredients:

- 3 cups skim milk
- 1 cup buckwheat grouts
- ¼ cup chia seeds
- 2 teaspoons vanilla extract
- 1/2 teaspoon ground cinnamon
- Pinch salt
- 1 cup water
- 1/2 cup unsalted pistachios
- 2 cups sliced fresh strawberries

- ¼ cup cacao nibs (optional)

Directions:
1. In a large bowl, stir together the milk, groats, chia seeds, vanilla, cinnamon, and salt. Cover and refrigerate overnight.
2. The next morning, transfer the soaked mixture to a medium pot and add the water. Bring to a boil over medium-high heat, reduce the heat to maintain a simmer, and cook for 10 to 12 minutes, until the buckwheat is tender and thickened.
3. Transfer to bowls and serve, topped with the pistachios, strawberries, and cacao nibs (if using).

Nutrition: Calories: 340; Total Fat: 8g; Saturated Fat: 1g; Protein: 15g; Carbs: 52g; Sugar: 14g; Fiber: 10g; Cholesterol: 4mg; Sodium: 140mg

4. Peach Muesli Bake

Preparation Time: 10 minutes
Cooking Time: 40 minutes
Servings: 8
Ingredients:
- Nonstick cooking spray
- 2 cups skim milk
- 1 1/2 cups rolled oats
- 1/2 cup chopped walnuts
- 1 large egg
- 2 tablespoons maple syrup
- 1 teaspoon ground cinnamon
- 1 teaspoon baking powder
- 1/2 teaspoon salt
- 2 to 3 peaches, sliced

Directions:
1. Preheat the oven to 375f. Spray a 9-inch square baking dish with cooking spray. Set aside.
2. In a large bowl, stir together the milk, oats, walnuts, egg, maple syrup, cinnamon, baking powder, and salt. Spread half the mixture in the prepared baking dish.

3. Place half the peaches in a single layer across the oat mixture.
4. Spread the remaining oat mixture over the top. Add the remaining peaches in a thin layer over the oats. Bake for 35 to 40 minutes, uncovered, until thickened and browned.
5. Cut into 8 squares and serve warm.

Nutrition: Calories: 138; Total Fat: 3g; Saturated Fat: 1g; Protein: 6g; Carbs: 22g; Sugar: 10g; Fiber: 3g; Cholesterol: 24mg; Sodium: 191mg

5. Steel-Cut Oatmeal Bowl With Fruit And Nuts

Preparation Time: 5 minutes
Cooking Time: 20 minutes
Servings: 4
Ingredients:

- 1 cup steel-cut oats
- 2 cups almond milk
- ¾ cup water
- 1 teaspoon ground cinnamon
- ¼ teaspoon salt
- 2 cups chopped fresh fruit, such as blueberries, strawberries, raspberries, or peaches
- 1/2 cup chopped walnuts
- ¼ cup chia seeds

Directions:

1. In a medium saucepan over medium-high heat, combine the oats, almond milk, water, cinnamon, and salt. Bring to a boil, reduce the heat to low, and simmer for 15 to 20 minutes, until the oats are softened and thickened.

2. Top each bowl with 1/2 cup of fresh fruit, 2 tablespoons of walnuts, and 1 tablespoon of chia seeds before serving.

Nutrition: Calories: 288; Total Fat: 11g; Saturated Fat: 1g; Protein: 10g; Carbs: 38g; Sugar: 7g; Fiber: 10g; Cholesterol: 0mg; Sodium: 329mg

Appetizer Recipes

6. Cheesy Broccoli Bites

Preparation Time: 10 minutes
Cooking Time: 25 minutes
Serving: 6
Ingredients:
- 2 tablespoons olive oil
- 2 heads broccoli, trimmed
- 1 egg
- 1/3 cup reduced-fat shredded Cheddar cheese
- 1 egg white
- ½ cup onion, chopped
- 1/3 cup bread crumbs
- ¼ teaspoon salt
- ¼ teaspoon black pepper

Directions:
1. Ready the oven at 400°F (205°C). Coat a large baking sheet with olive oil.

2. Arrange a colander in a saucepan, then place the broccoli in the colander. Pour the water into the saucepan to cover the bottom. Boil, then reduce the heat to low. Close and simmer for 6 minutes. Allow cooling for 10 minutes.

3. Blend broccoli and remaining ingredients in a food processor. Let sit for 10 minutes.

4. Make the bites: Drop 1 tablespoon of the mixture on the baking sheet. Repeat with the remaining mixture.

5. Bake in the preheated oven for 25 minutes. Flip the bites halfway through the cooking time.

6. Serve immediately.

Nutrition:100 Calories; 13g Carbohydrates; 3g Fiber

7. Easy Caprese Skewers

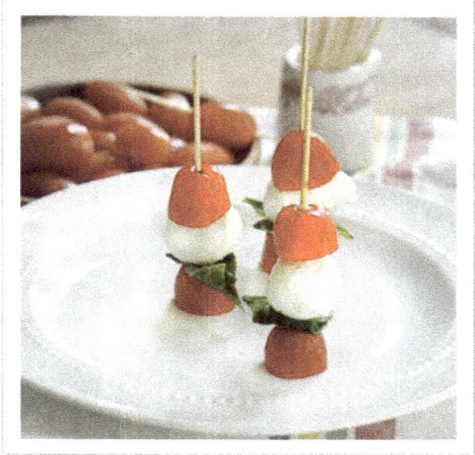

Preparation Time: 5 minutes

Cooking Time: 0 minute

Serving: 2

Ingredients:

- 12 cherry tomatoes
- 8 (1-inch) pieces Mozzarella cheese
- 12 basil leaves
- ¼ cup Italian Vinaigrette, for serving

Directions:

1. Thread the tomatoes, cheese, and bay leave alternatively through the skewers.
2. Place the skewers on a huge plate and baste with the Italian Vinaigrette. Serve immediately.

Nutrition: 230 Calories; 8.5g Carbohydrates; 1.9g Fiber

8. Grilled Tofu with Sesame Seeds

Preparation Time: 45 minutes
Cooking Time: 20 minutes
Serving: 6
Ingredients:

- 1½ tablespoons brown rice vinegar
- 1 scallion
- 1 tablespoon ginger root
- 1 tablespoon no-sugar-added applesauce
- 2 tablespoons naturally brewed soy sauce
- ¼ teaspoon dried red pepper flakes
- 2 teaspoons sesame oil, toasted
- 1 (14-ounce / 397-g) package extra-firm tofu
- 2 tablespoons fresh cilantro
- 1 teaspoon sesame seeds

Directions:

1. Combine the vinegar, scallion, ginger, applesauce, soy sauce, red pepper flakes, and sesame oil in a large bowl. Stir to mix well.
2. Dunk the tofu pieces in the bowl, then refrigerate to marinate for 30 minutes.

3. Preheat a grill pan over medium-high heat.

4. Place the tofu on the grill pan with tongs, reserve the marinade, then grill for 8 minutes or until the tofu is golden brown and have deep grilled marks on both sides. Flip the tofu halfway through the cooking time. You may need to work in batches to avoid overcrowding.

5. Transfer the tofu to a large plate and sprinkle with cilantro leaves and sesame seeds. Serve with the marinade alongside.

Nutrition: 90 Calories; 3g Carbohydrates; 1g Fiber

9. Kale Chips

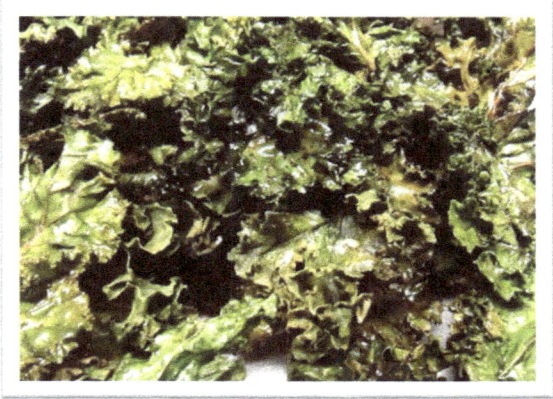

Preparation Time: 5 minutes

Cooking Time: 15 minutes

Serving: 1

Ingredients:

- ¼ teaspoon garlic powder
- Pinch cayenne to taste
- 1 tablespoon extra-virgin olive oil
- ½ teaspoon sea salt, or to taste
- 1 (8-ounce) bunch kale

Directions:

1. Prepare oven at 180°C. Line two baking sheets with parchment paper.
2. Toss the garlic powder, cayenne pepper, olive oil, and salt in a large bowl, then dunk the kale in the bowl.

3. Situate kale in a single layer on one of the baking sheets.

4. Arrange the sheet in the preheated oven and bake for 7 minutes. Remove the sheet from the oven and pour the kale into the single layer of the other baking sheet.

5. Move the sheet of kale back to the oven and bake for another 7 minutes.

6. Serve immediately.

Nutrition: 136 Calories; 3g Carbohydrates; 1.1g Fiber

10.   Simple Deviled Eggs

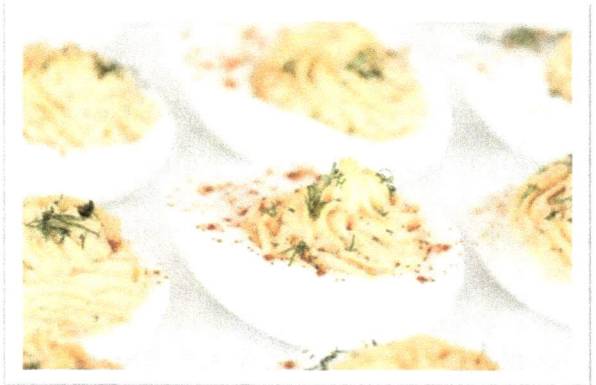

Preparation Time: 5 minutes

Cooking Time: 8 minutes

Serving: 12

Ingredients:

- 6 large eggs
- 1/8 teaspoon mustard powder
- 2 tablespoons light mayonnaise

Directions:

1. Sit the eggs in a saucepan, then pour in enough water to cover the egg. Bring to a boil, then boil the eggs for another 8 minutes. Turn off the heat and cover, then let sit for 15 minutes.
2. Transfer the boiled eggs to a pot of cold water and peel under the water.

3. Transfer the eggs to a large plate, then cut in half. Remove the egg yolks and place them in a bowl, then mash with a fork.

4. Add the mustard powder, mayo, salt, and pepper to the bowl of yolks, then stir to mix well.

5. Spoon the yolk mixture in the egg white on the plate. Serve immediately.

Nutrition: 45 Calories; 1g Carbohydrates; 0.9g Fiber

11. Sautéed Collard Greens and Cabbage

Preparation Time: 10 minutes
Cooking Time: 10 minutes
Serving: 8
Ingredients:

- 2 tablespoons extra-virgin olive oil
- 1 collard greens bunch
- ½ small green cabbage
- 6 garlic cloves
- 1 tablespoon low-sodium soy sauce

Directions:

1. Cook olive oil in a large skillet over medium-high heat.
2. Sauté the collard greens in the oil for about 2 minutes, or until the greens start to wilt.
3. Toss in the cabbage and mix well. Set to medium-low, cover, and cook for 5 to 7 minutes, stirring occasionally, or until the greens are softened.
4. Fold in the garlic and soy sauce and stir to combine. Cook for about 30 seconds more until fragrant.
5. Remove from the heat to a plate and serve.

Nutrition: 73 Calories; 5.9g Carbohydrates; 2.9g Fiber

12. Roasted Delicata Squash with Thyme

Preparation Time: 10 minutes
Cooking Time: 20 minutes
Serving: 4
Ingredients:

- 1 (1½-pound) Delicata squash
- 1 tablespoon extra-virgin olive oil
- ½ teaspoon dried thyme
- ¼ teaspoon salt
- ¼ teaspoon freshly ground black pepper

Directions:

1. Prep the oven to 400°F (205°C). Ready baking sheet with parchment paper and set aside.
2. Add the squash strips, olive oil, thyme, salt, and pepper in a large bowl, and toss until the squash strips are fully coated.
3. Place the squash strips on the prepared baking sheet in a single layer. Roast for about 20 minutes, flipping the strips halfway through.
4. Remove from the oven and serve on plates.

Nutrition: 78 Calories; 11.8g Carbohydrates; 2.1g Fiber

First Course Recipes

13. Blueberry and Chicken Salad

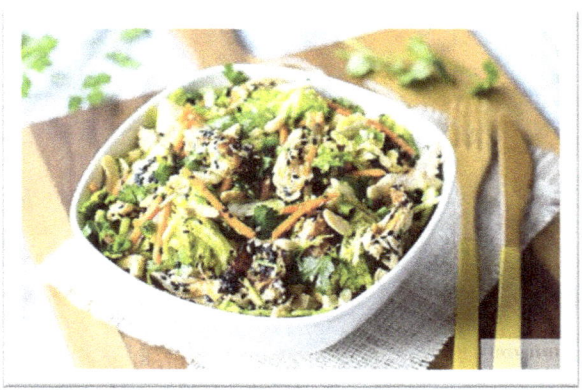

Preparation Time: 10 minutes

Cooking Time: 0 minute

Serving: 4

Ingredients:

- 2 cups chopped cooked chicken
- 1 cup fresh blueberries
- ¼ cup almonds
- 1 celery stalk
- ¼ cup red onion
- 1 tablespoon fresh basil
- 1 tablespoon fresh cilantro

- ½ cup plain, vegan mayonnaise
- ¼ teaspoon salt
- ¼ teaspoon freshly ground black pepper
- 8 cups salad greens

Directions:
1. Toss chicken, blueberries, almonds, celery, onion, basil, and cilantro.
2. Blend yogurt, salt, and pepper. Stir chicken salad to combine.
3. Situate 2 cups of salad greens on each of 4 plates and divide the chicken salad among the plates to serve.

Nutrition: 207 Calories; 11g Carbohydrates; 6g Sugars

14. Beef and Red Bean Chili

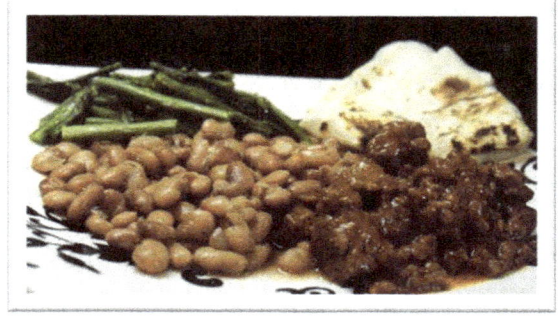

Preparation Time: 10 minutes
Cooking Time: 6 hours
Serving: 4
Ingredients:

- 1 cup dry red beans
- 1 tablespoon olive oil
- 2 pounds boneless beef chuck
- 1 large onion, coarsely chopped
- 1 (14 ounce) can beef broth
- 2 chipotle chili peppers in adobo sauce
- 2 teaspoons dried oregano, crushed
- 1 teaspoon ground cumin
- ½ teaspoon salt
- 1 (14.5 ounce) can tomatoes with mild green chilis

- 1 (15 ounce) can tomato sauce
- ¼ cup snipped fresh cilantro
- 1 medium red sweet pepper

Directions:

1. Rinse out the beans and place them into a Dutch oven or big saucepan, then add in water enough to cover them. Allow the beans to boil then drop the heat down. Simmer the beans without a cover for 10 minutes. Take off the heat and keep covered for an hour.

2. In a big frypan, heat up the oil upon medium-high heat, then cook onion and half the beef until they brown a bit over medium-high heat. Move into a 3 1/2- or 4-quart crockery cooker. Do this again with what's left of the beef. Add in tomato sauce, tomatoes (not drained), salt, cumin, oregano, adobo sauce, chipotle peppers, and broth, stirring to blend. Strain out and rinse beans and stir in the cooker.

3. Cook while covered on a low setting for around 10-12 hours or on high setting for 5-6 hours. Spoon the chili into bowls or mugs and top with sweet pepper and cilantro.

Nutrition: 288 Calories; 24g Carbohydrate; 5g Sugar

15. Berry Apple Cider

Preparation Time: 15 minutes
Cooking Time: 3 hours
Serving: 3
Ingredients:

- 4 cinnamon sticks, cut into 1-inch pieces
- 1½ teaspoons whole cloves
- 4 cups apple cider
- 4 cups low-calorie cranberry-raspberry juice drink
- 1 medium apple

Directions:

1. To make the spice bag, cut out a 6-inch square from double thick, pure cotton cheesecloth. Put in the cloves and cinnamon, then bring the corners up, tie it closed using a clean kitchen string that is pure cotton.
2. In a 3 1/2- 5-quart slow cooker, combine cranberry-raspberry juice, apple cider, and the spice bag.
3. Cook while covered over low heat setting for around 4-6 hours or on a high heat setting for 2-2 1/2 hours.

4. Throw out the spice bag. Serve right away or keep it warm while covered on warm or low-heat setting up to 2 hours, occasionally stirring. Garnish each serving with apples (thinly sliced).

Nutrition: 89 Calories; 22g Carbohydrate; 19g Sugar

16. Brunswick Stew

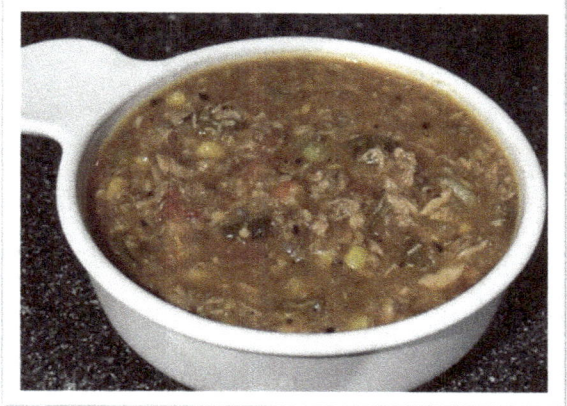

Preparation Time: 10 minutes
Cooking Time: 45 minutes
Serving: 3
Ingredients:

- 4 ounces diced salt pork
- 2 pounds chicken parts
- 8 cups water
- 3 potatoes, cubed
- 3 onions, chopped
- 1 (28 ounce) can whole peeled tomatoes
- 2 cups canned whole kernel corn
- 1 (10 ounce) package frozen lima beans

- 1 tablespoon Worcestershire sauce
- 1/2 teaspoon salt
- 1/4 teaspoon ground black pepper

Directions:
1. Mix and boil water, chicken and salt pork in a big pot on high heat. Lower heat to low. Cover then simmer until chicken is tender for 45 minutes.
2. Take out chicken. Let cool until easily handled. Take meat out. Throw out bones and skin. Chop meat to bite-sized pieces. Put back in the soup.
3. Add ground black pepper, salt, Worcestershire sauce, lima beans, corn, tomatoes, onions and potatoes. Mix well. Stir well and simmer for 1 hour, uncovered.

Nutrition: 368 Calories; 25.9g Carbohydrate; 27.9g Protein

Second Course Recipes

17. Cauliflower Rice with Chicken

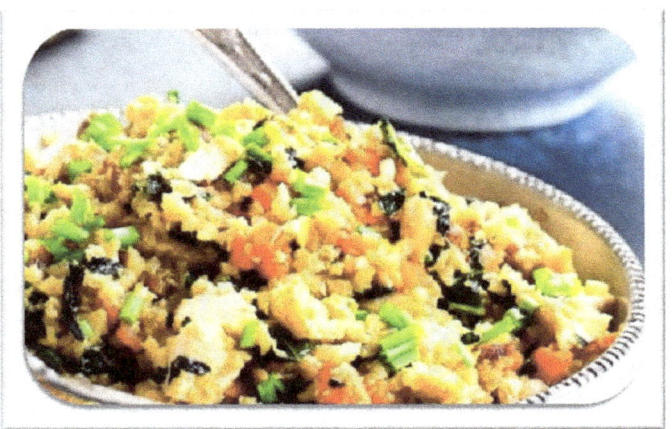

Preparation Time: 15 Minutes

Cooking Time: 15 Minutes

Servings: 4

Ingredients:

- 1/2 large cauliflower
- 3/4 cup cooked meat
- 1/2 bell pepper
- 1 carrot
- 2 ribs celery
- 1 tbsp. stir fry sauce (low carb)

- 1 tbsp. extra virgin olive oil
- Salt and pepper to taste

Directions:
1. Chop cauliflower in a processor to "rice." Place in a bowl.
2. Properly chop all vegetables in a food processor into thin slices.
3. Add cauliflower and other plants to WOK with heated oil. Fry until all veggies are tender.
4. Add chopped meat and sauce to the wok and fry 10 Minutes.
5. Serve

This dish is very mouth-watering!

Nutrition: Calories 200; Protein 10 g; Fat 12 g; Carbs 10 g

18. Turkey with Fried Eggs

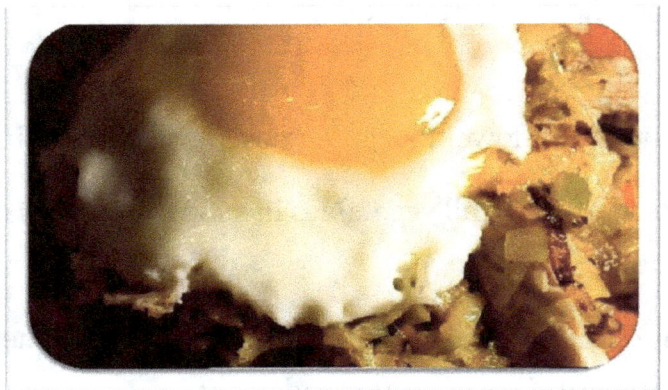

Preparation Time: 10 Minutes

Cooking Time: 20 Minutes

Servings: 4

Ingredients:

- 4 large potatoes
- 1 cooked turkey thigh
- 1 large onion (about 2 cups diced)
- butter
- Chile flakes
- 4 eggs
- salt to taste
- pepper to taste

Directions:
1. Rub the cold boiled potatoes on the coarsest holes of a box grater. Dice the turkey.
2. Cook the onion in as much unsalted butter as you feel comfortable with until it's just fragrant and translucent.
3. Add the rubbed potatoes and a cup of diced cooked turkey, salt and pepper to taste, and cook 20 Minutes.

Top each with a fried egg. Yummy!

Nutrition: Calories 170; Protein 19 g; Fat 7 g; Carbs 6 g

19. Sweet Potato, Kale, and White Bean Stew

Preparation Time: 15 minutes
Cooking Time: 25 minutes
Servings: 4
Ingredients:

- 1 (15-ounce) can low-sodium cannellini beans, rinsed and drained, divided
- 1 tablespoon olive oil
- 1 medium onion, chopped
- 2 garlic cloves, minced
- 2 celery stalks, chopped
- 3 medium carrots, chopped
- 2 cups low-sodium vegetable broth
- 1 teaspoon apple cider vinegar
- 2 medium sweet potatoes (about 1¼ pounds)
- 2 cups chopped kale
- 1 cup shelled edamame
- ¼ cup quinoa
- 1 teaspoon dried thyme
- 1/2 teaspoon cayenne pepper

- 1/2 teaspoon salt
- ¼ teaspoon freshly ground black pepper

Directions:

1. Put half the beans into a blender and blend until smooth. Set aside.

2. In a large soup pot over medium heat, heat the oil. When the oil is shining, include the onion and garlic, and cook until the onion softens and the garlic is sweet, about 3 minutes. Add the celery and carrots, and continue cooking until the vegetables soften, about 5 minutes.

3. Add the broth, vinegar, sweet potatoes, unblended beans, kale, edamame, and quinoa, and bring the mixture to a boil. Reduce the heat and simmer until the vegetables soften, about 10 minutes.

4. Add the blended beans, thyme, cayenne, salt, and black pepper, increase the heat to medium-high, and bring the mixture to a boil. Reduce the heat and simmer, uncovered, until the flavors combine, about 5 minutes.

5. Into each of 4 containers, scoop 1¾ cups of stew.

Nutrition: Calories: 373; Total Fat: 7g; Saturated Fat: 1g; Protein: 15g; Total Carbs: 65g; Fiber: 15g; Sugar: 13g; Sodium: 540mg

20. Slow Cooker Two-Bean Sloppy Joes

Preparation Time: 10 minutes
Cooking Time: 6 hours
Servings: 4
Ingredients:

- 1 (15-ounce) can low-sodium black beans
- 1 (15-ounce) can low-sodium pinto beans
- 1 (15-ounce) can no-salt-added diced tomatoes
- 1 medium green bell pepper, cored, seeded, and chopped
- 1 medium yellow onion, chopped
- ¼ cup low-sodium vegetable broth
- 2 garlic cloves, minced
- 2 servings (¼ cup) meal prep barbecue sauce or bottled barbecue sauce
- ¼ teaspoon salt
- ¼ teaspoon freshly ground black pepper
- 4 whole-wheat buns

Directions:

1. In a slow cooker, combine the black beans, pinto beans, diced tomatoes, bell pepper, onion, broth, garlic, meal prep barbecue sauce, salt, and black pepper. Stir the ingredients, then cover and cook on low for 6 hours.

2. Into each of 4 containers, spoon 1¼ cups of sloppy joe mix. Serve with 1 whole-wheat bun.

3. Storage: place airtight containers in the refrigerator for up to 1 week. To freeze, place freezer-safe containers in the freezer for up to 2 months. To defrost, refrigerate overnight. To reheat individual portions, microwave uncovered on high for 2 to 21/2 minutes. Alternatively, reheat the entire dish in a saucepan on the stove top. Bring the sloppy joes to a boil, then reduce the heat and simmer until heated through, 10 to 15 minutes. Serve with a whole-wheat bun.

Nutrition: Calories: 392; Total Fat: 3g; Saturated Fat: 0g; Protein: 17g; Total Carbs: 79g; Fiber: 19g; Sugar: 15g; Sodium: 759mg

21. Lighter Eggplant Parmesan

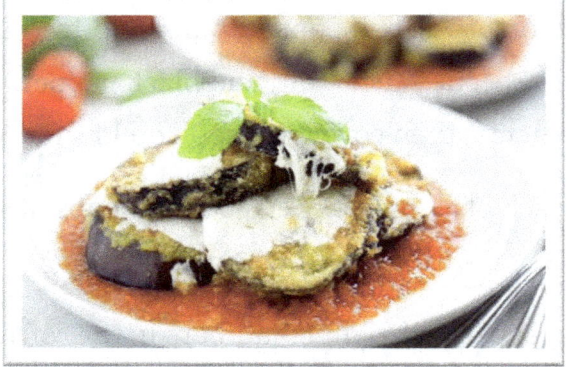

Preparation Time: 15 minutes

Cooking Time: 35 minutes

Servings: 4

Ingredients:

- Nonstick cooking spray
- 3 eggs, beaten
- 1 tablespoon dried parsley
- 2 teaspoons ground oregano
- 1/8 teaspoon freshly ground black pepper
- 1 cup panko bread crumbs, preferably whole-wheat
- 1 large eggplant (about 2 pounds)
- 5 servings (21/2 cups) chunky tomato sauce or jarred low-sodium tomato sauce

- 1 cup part-skim mozzarella cheese
- ¼ cup grated parmesan cheese

Directions:

1. Preheat the oven to 450f. Coat a baking sheet with cooking spray.
2. In a medium bowl, whisk together the eggs, parsley, oregano, and pepper.
3. Pour the panko into a separate medium bowl.
4. Slice the eggplant into ¼-inch-thick slices. Dip each slice of eggplant into the egg mixture, shaking off the excess. Then dredge both sides of the eggplant in the panko bread crumbs. Place the coated eggplant on the prepared baking sheet, leaving a 1/2-inch space between each slice.
5. Bake for about 15 minutes until soft and golden brown. Remove from the oven and set aside to slightly cool.
6. Pour 1/2 cup of chunky tomato sauce on the bottom of an 8-by-15-inch baking dish. Using a spatula or the back of a spoon spread the tomato sauce evenly. Place half the slices of cooked eggplant, slightly overlapping, in the dish, and top with 1 cup of chunky tomato sauce, 1/2 cup of mozzarella and 2 tablespoons of grated parmesan. Repeat the layer, ending with the cheese.

7. Bake uncovered for 20 minutes until the cheese is bubbling and slightly browned.

8. Remove from the oven and allow cooling for 15 minutes before dividing the eggplant equally into 4 separate containers.

Nutrition: Calories: 333; Total Fat: 14g; Saturated Fat: 6g; Protein: 20g; Total Carbs: 35g; Fiber: 11g; Sugar: 15g; Sodium: 994mg

22. Coconut-Lentil Curry

Preparation Time: 15 minutes
Cooking Time: 35 minutes
Servings: 4
Ingredients:

- 1 tablespoon olive oil
- 1 medium yellow onion, chopped
- 1 garlic clove, minced
- 1 medium red bell pepper, diced
- 1 (15-ounce) can green or brown lentils, rinsed and drained
- 2 medium sweet potatoes, washed, peeled, and cut into bite-size chunks (about 1¼ pounds)
- 1 (15-ounce) can no-salt-added diced tomatoes
- 2 tablespoons tomato paste
- 4 teaspoons curry powder
- 1/8 teaspoon ground cloves
- 1 (15-ounce) can light coconut milk
- ¼ teaspoon salt

- 2 pieces whole-wheat naan bread, halved, or 4 slices crusty bread

Directions:

1. In a large saucepan over medium heat, heat the olive oil. When the oil is shimmering, add both the onion and garlic and cook until the onion softens and the garlic is sweet, for about 3 minutes.

2. Add the bell pepper and continue cooking until it softens, about 5 minutes more. Add the lentils, sweet potatoes, tomatoes, tomato paste, curry powder, and cloves, and bring the mixture to a boil. Reduce the heat to medium-low, cover, and simmer until the potatoes are softened, about 20 minutes.

3. Add the coconut milk and salt, and return to a boil. Reduce the heat and simmer until the flavors combine, about 5 minutes.

4. Into each of 4 containers, spoon 2 cups of curry.

5. Enjoy each serving with half of a piece of naan bread or 1 slice of crusty bread.

Nutrition: Calories: 559; Total Fat: 16g; Saturated Fat: 7g; Protein: 16g; Total Carbs: 86g; Fiber: 16g; Sugar: 18g; Sodium: 819mg

Side Dish Recipes

23.   Brussels Sprouts

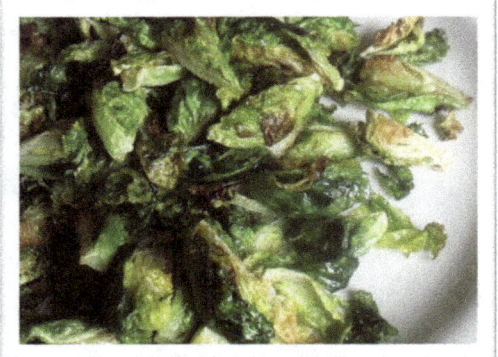

Preparation Time: 5 minutes

Cooking Time: 3 minutes

Servings: 5

Ingredients:

- 1 tsp. extra-virgin olive oil
- 1 lb. halved Brussels sprouts
- 3 tbsps. apple cider vinegar
- 3 tbsps. gluten-free tamari soy sauce
- 3 tbsps. chopped sun-dried tomatoes

Directions:

1. Select the "Sauté" function on your Instant Pot, add oil and allow the pot to get hot.
2. Cancel the "Sauté" function and add the Brussels sprouts.
3. Stir well and allow the sprouts to cook in the residual heat for 2-3 minutes.
4. Add the tamari soy sauce and vinegar, and then stir.
5. Cover the Instant Pot, sealing the pressure valve by pointing it to "Sealing."
6. Select the "Manual, High Pressure" setting and cook for 3 minutes.
7. Once the cook cycle is done, do a quick pressure release, and then stir in the chopped sun-dried tomatoes.
8. Serve immediately.

Nutrition: 62 Calories; 10g Carbohydrates; 1g Fat

24. Garlic and Herb Carrots

Preparation Time: 2 minutes
Cooking Time: 18 minutes
Servings: 3
Ingredients:
- 2 tbsps. butter
- 1 lb. baby carrots
- 1 cup water
- 1 tsp. fresh thyme or oregano
- 1 tsp. minced garlic
- Black pepper
- Coarse sea salt

Directions:
1. Fill water to the inner pot of the Instant Pot, and then put in a steamer basket.
2. Layer the carrots into the steamer basket.
3. Close and seal the lid, with the pressure vent in the "Sealing" position.
4. Select the "Steam" setting and cook for 2 minutes on high pressure.
5. Quick release the pressure and then carefully remove the steamer basket with the steamed carrots, discarding the water.

6. Add butter to the inner pot of the Instant Pot and allow it to melt on the "Sauté" function.
7. Add garlic and sauté for 30 seconds, and then add the carrots. Mix well.
8. Stir in the fresh herbs, and cook for 2-3 minutes.
9. Season with salt and black pepper, and the transfer to a serving bowl.
10. Serve warm and enjoy!

Nutrition: 122 Calories; 12g Carbohydrates; 7g Fat

25. Cilantro Lime Drumsticks

Preparation Time: 5 minutes
Cooking Time: 15 minutes
Servings: 6
Ingredients:

- 1 tbsp. olive oil
- 6 chicken drumsticks
- 4 minced garlic cloves
- ½ cup low-sodium chicken broth
- 1 tsp. cayenne pepper
- 1 tsp. crushed red peppers
- 1 tsp. fine sea salt
- Juice of 1 lime

To Serve:

- 2 tbsp. chopped cilantro
- Extra lime zest

Directions:

1. Pour olive oil to the Instant Pot and set it on the "Sauté" function.
2. Once the oil is hot adding the chicken drumsticks, and season them well.

3. Using tongs, stir the drumsticks and brown the drumsticks for 2 minutes per side.
4. Add the lime juice, fresh cilantro, and chicken broth to the pot.
5. Lock and seal the lid, turning the pressure valve to "Sealing."
6. Cook the drumsticks on the "Manual, High Pressure" setting for 9 minutes.
7. Once done let the pressure release naturally.
8. Carefully transfer the drumsticks to an aluminum-foiled baking sheet and broil them in the oven for 3-5 minutes until golden brown.
9. Serve warm, garnished with more cilantro and lime zest.

Nutrition: 480 Calories; 3.3g Carbohydrates; 29g Fat

26. Eggplant Spread

Preparation Time: 5 minutes
Cooking Time: 18 minutes
Servings: 5
Ingredients:

- 4 tbsps. extra-virgin olive oil
- 2 lbs. eggplant
- 4 skin-on garlic cloves
- ½ cup water
- ¼ cup pitted black olives
- 3 sprigs fresh thyme
- Juice of 1 lemon
- 1 tbsp. tahini
- 1 tsp. sea salt
- Fresh extra-virgin olive oil

Directions:

1. Peel the eggplant in alternating stripes, leaving some areas with skin and some with no skin.
2. Slice into big chunks and layer at the bottom of your Instant Pot.

3. Add olive oil to the pot, and on the "Sauté" function, fry and caramelize the eggplant on one side, about 5 minutes.
4. Add in the garlic cloves with the skin on.
5. Flip over the eggplant and then add in the remaining uncooked eggplant chunks, salt, and water.
6. Close the lid, ensure the pressure release valve is set to "Sealing."
7. Cook for 5 minutes on the "Manual, High Pressure" setting.
8. Once done, carefully open the pot by quick releasing the pressure through the steam valve.
9. Discard most of the brown cooking liquid.
10. Remove the garlic cloves and peel them.
11. Add the lemon juice, tahini, cooked and fresh garlic cloves and pitted black olives to the pot.
12. Using a hand-held immersion blender, process all the ingredients until smooth.
13. Pour out the spread into a serving dish and season with fresh thyme, whole black olives and some extra-virgin olive oil, prior to serving.

Nutrition: 155 Calories; 16.8g Carbohydrates; 11.7g Fat

27. Carrot Hummus

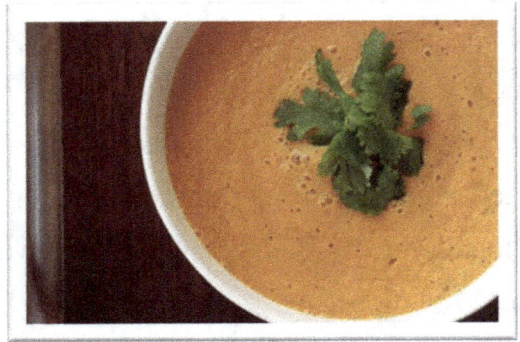

Preparation Time: 15 minutes
Cooking Time: 10 minutes
Servings: 2
Ingredients:

- 1 chopped carrot
- 2 oz. cooked chickpeas
- 1 tsp. lemon juice
- 1 tsp. tahini
- 1 tsp. fresh parsley

Directions:

1. Place the carrot and chickpeas in your Instant Pot.
2. Add a cup of water, seal, cook for 10 minutes on Stew.
3. Depressurize naturally. Blend with the remaining ingredients.

Nutrition: 58 Calories; 8g Carbohydrates; 2g Fat

28. Vegetable Rice Pilaf

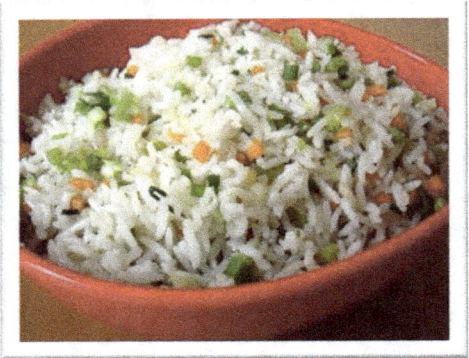

Preparation Time: 5 minutes

Cooking Time: 25 minutes

Servings: 6

Ingredients:

- 1 tablespoon olive oil
- ½ medium yellow onion, diced
- 1 cup uncooked long-grain brown rice
- 2 cloves minced garlic
- ½ teaspoon dried basil
- Salt and pepper
- 2 cups fat-free chicken broth
- 1 cup frozen mixed veggies

Directions:
1. Cook oil in a large skillet over medium heat.
2. Add the onion and sauté for 3 minutes until translucent.
3. Stir in the rice and cook until lightly toasted.
4. Add the garlic, basil, salt, and pepper then stir to combined.
5. Stir in the chicken broth then bring to a boil.
6. Decrease heat and simmer, covered, for 10 minutes.
7. Stir in the frozen veggies then cover and cook for another 10 minutes until heated through. Serve hot.

Nutrition: 90 Calories; 12.6g Carbohydrates; 2.2g Fiber

29.   Curry Roasted Cauliflower Florets

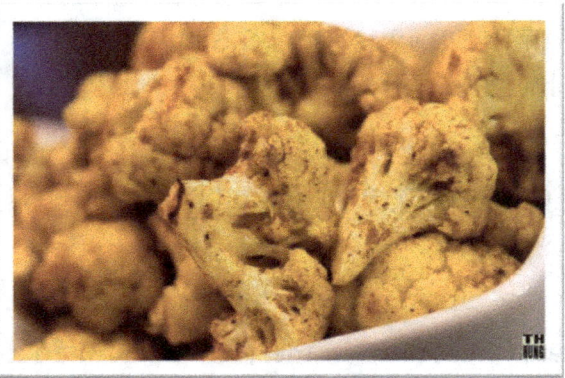

Preparation Time: 5 minutes
Cooking Time: 25 minutes
Servings: 6
Ingredients:

- 8 cups cauliflower florets
- 2 tablespoons olive oil
- 1 teaspoon curry powder
- ½ teaspoon garlic powder
- Salt and pepper

Directions:

1. Prep the oven to 425°F and line a baking sheet with foil.
2. Toss the cauliflower with the olive oil and spread on the baking sheet.

3. Sprinkle with curry powder, garlic powder, salt, and pepper.
4. Roast for 25 minutes or until just tender. Serve hot.

Nutrition: 75 Calories; 7.4g Carbohydrates; 3.5g Fiber

Soups & Stews

30. Dill Celery Soup

Preparation Time: 10 minutes

Cooking Time: 30 minutes

Servings: 4

Ingredients:

- 6 cups celery stalk, chopped
- 2 cups filtered alkaline water
- 1 medium onion, chopped
- 1/2 tsp. dill
- 1 cup of coconut milk
- 1/4 tsp. sea salt

Directions:

1. Combine all elements into the direct pot and mix fine.
2. Cover pot with lid and select soup mode it takes 30 minutes.
3. Release pressure using the quick release Directions: than open lid carefully.
4. Blend the soup utilizing a submersion blender until smooth.

5. Stir well and serve.

Nutrition: Calories 193; Fat 15.3 g; Carbohydrates 10.9 g; Protein 5.2 g; Sugar 5.6 g; Cholesterol 0 mg

31. Creamy Avocado-Broccoli Soup

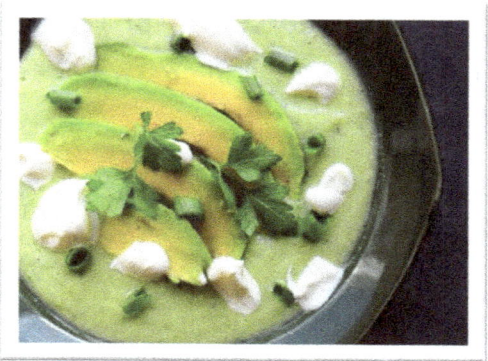

Preparation Time: 10 minutes

Cooking Time: 15 minutes

Servings: 1-2

Ingredients:
- 2-3 flowers broccoli
- 1 small avocado
- 1 yellow onion
- 1 green or red pepper
- 1 celery stalk
- 2 cups vegetable broth (yeast-free)
- Celtic Sea Salt to taste

Directions:

1. Warmth vegetable stock (don't bubble). Include hacked onion and broccoli, and warm for a few minutes. At that point put in blender, include the avocado, pepper and celery and Blend until the soup is smooth (include some more water whenever wanted). Flavor and serve warm. Delicious!!

Nutrition: Calories: 60g; Carbohydrates: 11g; Fat: 2 g; Protein: 2g

32.   Fresh Garden Vegetable Soup

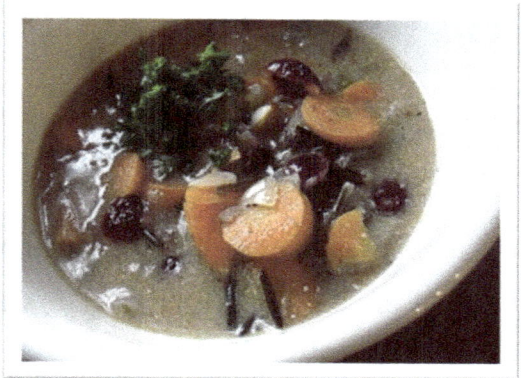

Preparation Time: 7 minutes

Cooking Time: 20 minutes

Servings: 1-2

Ingredients:

- 2 huge carrots
- 1 little zucchini
- 1 celery stem
- 1 cup of broccoli
- 3 stalks of asparagus
- 1 yellow onion
- 1 quart of (antacid) water
- 4-5 tsps. Of sans yeast vegetable stock

- 1 tsp. new basil
- 2 tsps. Ocean salt to taste

Directions:

1. Put water in pot, include the vegetable stock just as the onion and bring to bubble.
2. In the meantime, cleave the zucchini, the broccoli and the asparagus, and shred the carrots and the celery stem in a food processor.
3. When the water is bubbling, it would be ideal if you turn off the oven as we would prefer not to heat up the vegetables. Simply put them all in the high temp water and hold up until the vegetables arrive at wanted delicacy.
4. Permit to cool somewhat, at that point put all fixings into blender and blend until you get a thick, smooth consistency.

Nutrition: Calories: 43; Carbohydrates: 7g; Fat: 1 g

33.   Raw Some Gazpacho Soup

Preparation Time: 7 minutes
Cooking Time: 3 hours
Servings: 3-4
Ingredients:

- 500g tomatoes
- 1 small cucumber
- 1 red pepper
- 1 onion
- 2 cloves of garlic
- 1 small chili
- 1 quart of water (preferably alkaline water)
- 4 tbsp. cold-pressed olive oil
- Juice of one fresh lemon
- 1 dash of cayenne pepper
- Sea salt to taste

Directions:

1. Remove the skin of the cucumber and cut all vegetables in large pieces.

2. Put all Ingredients except the olive oil in a blender and mix until smooth.

3. Add the olive oil and mix again until oil is emulsified.

4. Put the soup in the fridge and chill for at least 2 hours (soup should be served ice cold).

5. Add some salt and pepper to taste, mix, place the soup in bowls, garnish with chopped scallions, cucumbers, tomatoes and peppers and enjoy!

Nutrition: Calories: 39; Carbohydrates: 8g; Fat: 0.5 g; Protein: 0.2g

34. Alkaline Carrot Soup with Fresh Mushrooms

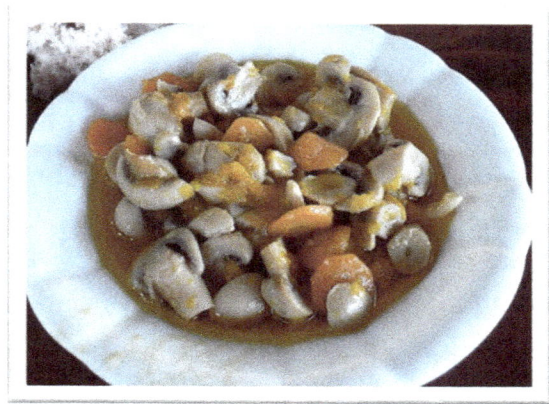

Preparation Time: 10 minutes
Cooking Time: 20 minutes
Servings: 1-2
Ingredients:
- 4 mid-sized carrots
- 4 mid-sized potatoes
- 10 enormous new mushrooms (champignons or chanterelles)
- 1/2 white onion
- 2 tbsp. olive oil (cold squeezed, additional virgin)
- 3 cups vegetable stock
- 2 tbsp. parsley, new and cleaved

- Salt and new white pepper

Directions:

1. Wash and strip carrots and potatoes and dice them.

2. Warm up vegetable stock in a pot on medium heat. Cook carrots and potatoes for around 15 minutes. Meanwhile finely shape onion and braise them in a container with olive oil for around 3 minutes.

3. Wash mushrooms, slice them to wanted size and add to the container, cooking approx. an additional 5 minutes, blending at times. Blend carrots, vegetable stock and potatoes, and put substance of the skillet into pot.

4. When nearly done, season with parsley, salt and pepper and serve hot. Appreciate this alkalizing soup!

Nutrition: Calories: 75; Carbohydrates: 13g; Fat: 1.8g; Protein: 1 g

Desserts

35. Peanut Butter Cups

Preparation Time: 5 minutes
Cooking Time: 10 minutes
Servings: 4
Ingredients:

- 1 packet plain gelatin
- ¼ cup sugar substitute
- 2 cups nonfat cream
- ½ teaspoon vanilla
- ¼ cup low-fat peanut butter
- 2 tablespoons unsalted peanuts, chopped

Directions:
1. Mix gelatin, sugar substitute and cream in a pan.
2. Let sit for 5 minutes.
3. Place over medium heat and cook until gelatin has been dissolved.
4. Stir in vanilla and peanut butter.
5. Pour into custard cups. Chill for 3 hours.
6. Top with the peanuts and serve.

Nutrition: 171 Calories; 21g Carbohydrate; 6.8g Protein

36.   Fruit Pizza

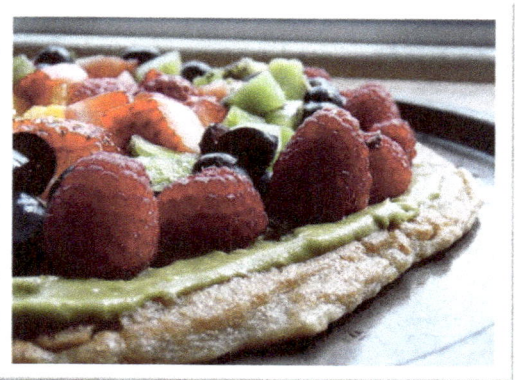

Preparation Time: 5 minutes
Cooking Time: 10 minutes
Servings: 4
Ingredients:

- 1 teaspoon maple syrup
- ¼ teaspoon vanilla extract
- ½ cup coconut milk yogurt
- 2 round slices watermelon
- ½ cup blackberries, sliced
- ½ cup strawberries, sliced
- 2 tablespoons coconut flakes (unsweetened)

Directions:

1. Mix maple syrup, vanilla and yogurt in a bowl.

2. Spread the mixture on top of the watermelon slice.
3. Top with the berries and coconut flakes.

Nutrition: 70 Calories; 14.6g Carbohydrate; 1.2g Protein

37. Choco Peppermint Cake

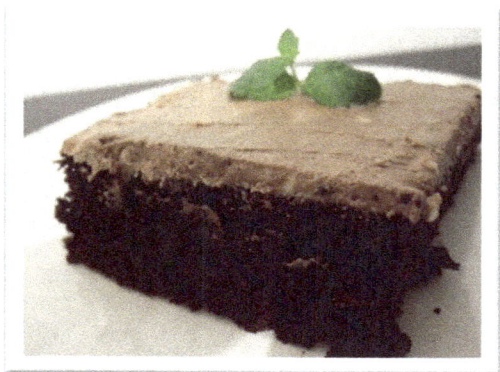

Preparation Time: 5 minutes
Cooking Time: 10 minutes
Servings: 4
Ingredients:
- Cooking spray
- 1/3 cup oil
- 15 oz. package chocolate cake mix
- 3 eggs, beaten
- 1 cup water
- ¼ teaspoon peppermint extract

Directions:
1. Spray slow cooker with oil.
2. Mix all the ingredients in a bowl.

3. Use an electric mixer on medium speed setting to mix ingredients for 2 minutes.
4. Pour mixture into the slow cooker.
5. Cover the pot and cook on low for 3 hours.
6. Let cool before slicing and serving.

Nutrition: 185 Calories; 27g Carbohydrate; 3.8g Protein

38.   Roasted Mango

Preparation Time: 5 minutes
Cooking Time: 10 minutes
Servings: 4
Ingredients:
- 2 mangoes, sliced
- 2 teaspoons crystallized ginger, chopped
- 2 teaspoons orange zest
- 2 tablespoons coconut flakes (unsweetened)

Directions:
1. Preheat your oven to 350 degrees F.
2. Add mango slices in custard cups.
3. Top with the ginger, orange zest and coconut flakes.
4. Bake in the oven for 10 minutes.

Nutrition: 89 Calories; 20g Carbohydrate; 0.8g Protein

39. Roasted Plums

Preparation Time: 5 minutes
Cooking Time: 10 minutes
Servings: 4
Ingredients:
- Cooking spray
- 6 plums, sliced
- ½ cup pineapple juice (unsweetened)
- 1 tablespoon brown sugar
- 2 tablespoons brown sugar
- ¼ teaspoon ground cardamom
- ½ teaspoon ground cinnamon
- 1/8 teaspoon ground cumin

Directions:
1. Combine all the ingredients in a baking pan.
2. Roast in the oven at 450 degrees F for 20 minutes.

Nutrition: 102 Calories; 18.7g Carbohydrate; 2g Protein

40.   Figs with Honey & Yogurt

Preparation Time: 5 minutes

Cooking Time: 10 minutes

Servings: 4

Ingredients:

- ½ teaspoon vanilla
- 8 oz. nonfat yogurt
- 2 figs, sliced
- 1 tablespoon walnuts, chopped and toasted
- 2 teaspoons honey

Directions:
1. Stir vanilla into yogurt.
2. Mix well.
3. Top with the figs and sprinkle with walnuts.
4. Drizzle with honey and serve.

Nutrition: 157 Calories; 24g Carbohydrate; 7g Protein

41. Flourless Chocolate Cake

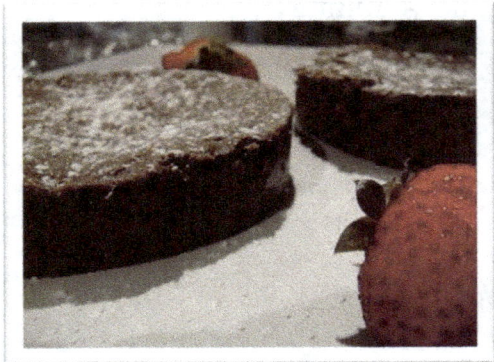

Preparation Time: 10 minutes

Cooking Time: 45 minutes

Servings: 6

Ingredients:
- ½ Cup of stevia
- 12 Ounces of unsweetened baking chocolate
- 2/3 Cup of ghee
- 1/3 Cup of warm water
- ¼ Teaspoon of salt
- 4 Large pastured eggs
- 2 Cups of boiling water

Directions:
1. Line the bottom of a 9-inch pan of a spring form with a parchment paper.

2. Heat the water in a small pot; then add the salt and the stevia over the water until wait until the mixture becomes completely dissolved.
3. Melt the baking chocolate into a double boiler or simply microwave it for about 30 seconds.
4. Mix the melted chocolate and the butter in a large bowl with an electric mixer.
5. Beat in your hot mixture; then crack in the egg and whisk after adding each of the eggs.
6. Pour the obtained mixture into your prepared spring form tray.
7. Wrap the spring form tray with a foil paper.
8. Place the spring form tray in a large cake tray and add boiling water right to the outside; make sure the depth doesn't exceed 1 inch.
9. Bake the cake into the water bath for about 45 minutes at a temperature of about 350 F.
10. Remove the tray from the boiling water and transfer to a wire to cool.
11. Let the cake chill for an overnight in the refrigerator.

<u>*Nutrition:*</u> 295 Calories; 6g Carbohydrates; 4g Fiber

42. Lava Cake

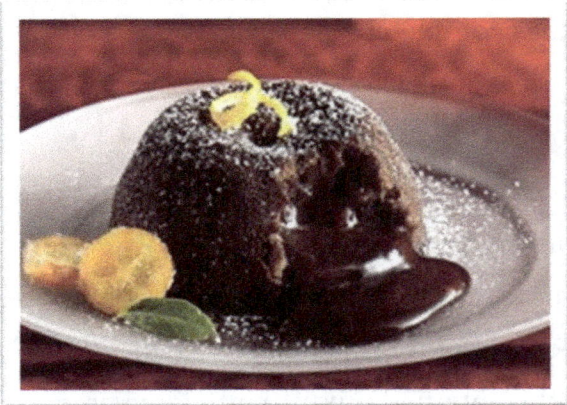

Preparation Time: 10 minutes
Cooking Time: 10 minutes
Servings: 2
Ingredients:

- 2 Oz of dark chocolate; you should at least use chocolate of 85% cocoa solids
- 1 Tablespoon of super-fine almond flour
- 2 Oz of unsalted almond butter
- 2 Large eggs

Directions:

1. Heat your oven to a temperature of about 350 Fahrenheit.
2. Grease 2 heat proof ramekins with almond butter.

3. Now, melt the chocolate and the almond butter and stir very well.
4. Beat the eggs very well with a mixer.
5. Add the eggs to the chocolate and the butter mixture and mix very well with almond flour and the swerve; then stir.
6. Pour the dough into 2 ramekins.
7. Bake for about 9 to 10 minutes.
8. Turn the cakes over plates and serve with pomegranate seeds!

Nutrition: 459 Calories; 3.5g Carbohydrates; 0.8g Fiber

Juice and Smoothie Recipes

43. Dandelion Avocado Smoothie

Preparation Time: 15 minutes

Cooking Time: 0

Servings: 1

Ingredients:

- One cup of Dandelion
- One Orange (juiced)
- Coconut water
- One Avocado
- One key lime (juice)

Directions:

1. In a high-speed blender until smooth, blend Ingredients.

Nutrition: Calories: 160; Fat: 15 g; Carbohydrates: 9 g; Protein: 2 g

44. Amaranth Greens and Avocado Smoothie

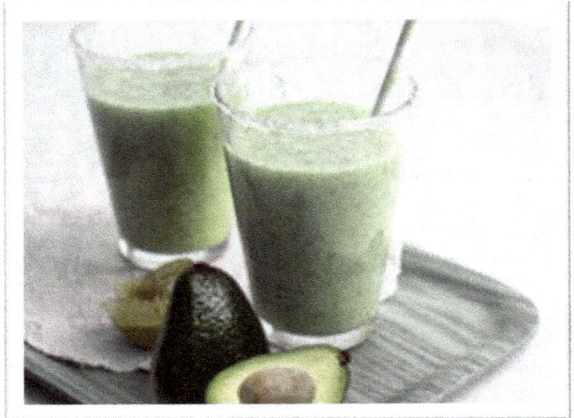

Preparation Time: 15 minutes
Cooking Time: 0
Servings: 1
Ingredients:

- One key lime (juice).

- Two sliced apples (seeded).

- Half avocado.

- Two cupsful of amaranth greens.

- Two cupsful of watercress.

- One cupful of water.

Directions:

1. Add the whole recipes together and transfer them into the blender. Blend thoroughly until smooth.

Nutrition: Calories: 160; Fat: 15 g; Carbohydrates: 9 g; Protein: 2 g

45. Lettuce, Orange and Banana Smoothie

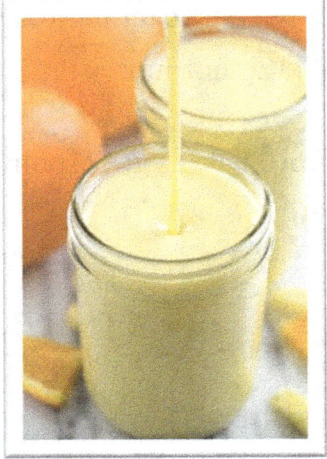

Preparation Time: 15 minutes

Cooking Time: 0

Servings: 1

Ingredients:

- One and a half cupsful of fresh lettuce.
- One large banana.
- One cup of mixed berries of your choice.
- One juiced orange.

Directions:
1. First, add the orange juice to your blender.
2. Add the remaining recipes and blend thoroughly.
3. Enjoy the rest of your day.

Nutrition: Calories: 252.1; Protein: 4.1 g

46. Delicious Elderberry Smoothie

Preparation Time: 15 minutes
Cooking Time: 0
Servings: 1
Ingredients:
- One cupful of Elderberry
- One cupful of Cucumber
- One large apple
- A quarter cupful of water

Directions:
1. Add the whole recipes together into a blender. Grind very well until they are uniformly smooth and enjoy.

Nutrition: Calories: 106; Carbohydrates: 26.68

47. Peaches Zucchini Smoothie

Preparation Time: 15 minutes
Cooking Time: 0
Servings: 1
Ingredients:

- A half cupful of squash.
- A half cupful of peaches.
- A quarter cupful of coconut water.
- A half cupful of Zucchini.

Directions:
1. Add the whole recipes together into a blender and blend until smooth and serve.

Nutrition: 55 Calories; 0g Fat; 2g Of Protein; 10mg Sodium; 14 G Carbohydrate; 2g Of Fiber

48. Ginger Orange and Strawberry Smoothie

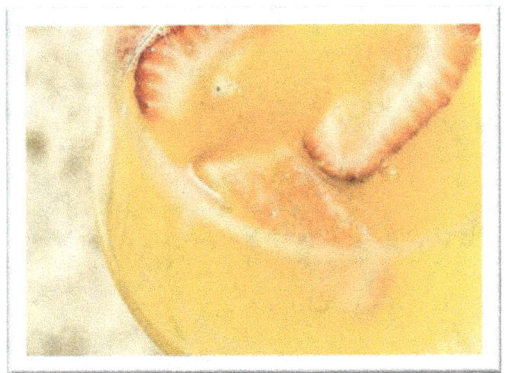

Preparation Time: 15 minutes

Cooking Time: 0

Servings: 1

Ingredients:

- One cup of strawberry.
- One large orange (juice).
- One large banana.
- Quarter small sized ginger (peeled and sliced).

Directions:

2. Transfer the orange juice to a clean blender.
3. Add the remaining recipes and blend thoroughly until smooth.

4. Enjoy. Wow! You have ended the 9th day of your weight loss and detox journey.

<u>Nutrition</u>: 32 Calories; 0.3g Fat; 2g Of Protein; 10mg Sodium; 14g Carbohydrate; Water; 2g Of Fiber.

49. Kale Parsley and Chia Seeds Detox Smoothie

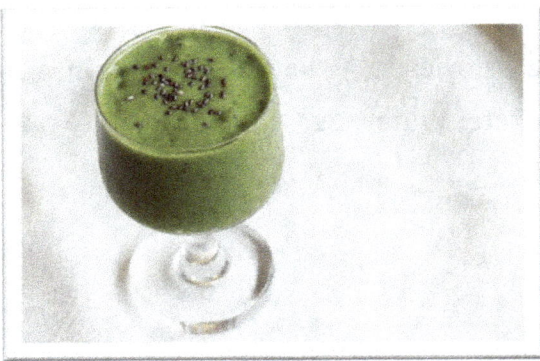

Preparation Time: 15 minutes

Cooking Time: 0

Servings: 1

Ingredients:

- Three tbsp. chia seeds (grounded).
- One cupful of water.
- One sliced banana.
- One pear (chopped).
- One cupful of organic kale.
- One cupful of parsley.
- Two tbsp. of lemon juice.
- A dash of cinnamon.

Directions:

1. Add the whole recipes together into a blender and pour the water before blending. Blend at high speed until smooth and enjoy.

   You may or may not place it in the refrigerator depending on how hot or cold the weather appears.

Nutrition: 75 calories; 1g fat; 5g protein; 10g fiber

50. Watermelon Limenade

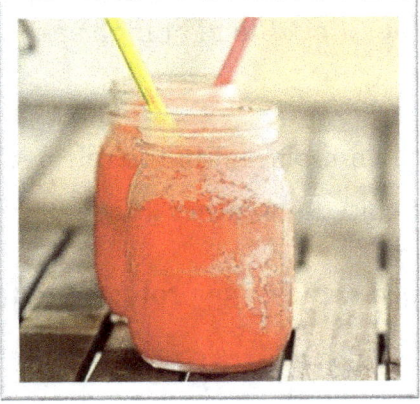

Preparation Time: 5 Minutes
Cooking Time: 0 minutes
Servings: 6

When it comes to refreshing summertime drinks, lemonade is always near the top of the list. This Watermelon "Limenade" is perfect for using up leftover watermelon or for those early fall days when stores and farmers are almost giving them away. You can also substitute 4 cups of ice for the cold water to create a delicious summertime slushy.

Ingredients:

- 4 cups diced watermelon
- 4 cups cold water
- 2 tablespoons freshly squeezed lemon juice
- 1 tablespoon freshly squeezed lime juice

Directions:

1. In a blender, combine the watermelon, water, lemon juice, and lime juice, and blend for 1 minute.

2. Strain the contents through a fine-mesh sieve or nut-milk bag. Serve chilled. Store in the refrigerator for up to 3 days.

SERVING TIP: Slice up a few lemon or lime wedges to serve with your Watermelon Limenade, or top it with a few fresh mint leaves to give it an extra-crisp, minty flavor.

Nutrition: Calories: 60

Conclusion

Being diagnosed with diabetes will bring some major changes in your lifestyle. From the time you are diagnosed with it, it would always be a constant battle with food. You need to become a lot more careful with your food choices and the quantity that you ate. Every meal will feel like a major effort. You will be planning every day for the whole week, well in advance. Depending upon the type of food you ate, you have to keep checking your blood sugar levels. You may get used to taking long breaks between meals and staying away from snacks between dinner and breakfast.

Managing diabetes can be a very, very stressful ordeal. But now, those days are gone!

Diabetes can occur at any age. However, being too young or too old means your body is not in its best form, and therefore, this increases the risk of developing diabetes.

If you start to notice you are prediabetic or getting overweight, etc., there is always something you can do to modify the situation. Recent studies show that developing healthy eating habits and following diets that are low in carbs, losing excess weight, and leading an active lifestyle can help to protect you from developing diabetes, especially diabetes type 2, by minimizing the risk factors of developing the disorder.

www.ingramcontent.com/pod-product-compliance
Lightning Source LLC
Chambersburg PA
CBHW070932080526
44589CB00013B/1486